Six Key Steps to Making a Dementia Friendly Church

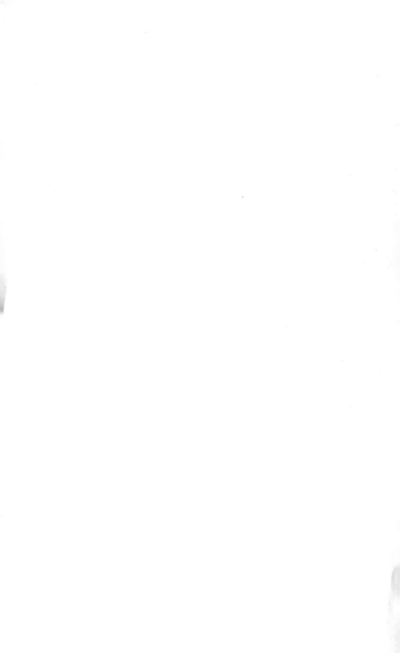

Six Key Steps
to Making a
Dementia
Friendly
Church

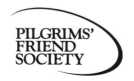

PILGRIMS'
FRIEND
SOCIETY

Six Key Steps to Making a Dementia Friendly Church

Proven Principles drawn from real life experience

Copyright © July 2014 Pilgrims' Friend Society.

Revised and reprinted 2020

A catalogue record for this book is available from the British Library.

ISBN 978-0-9930148-0-2

Designed and typeset by: Pete Barnsley (CreativeHoot.com)

Printed and bound by CPI Group (UK) Ltd, Croydon, CR0 4YY

First published in the UK in 2014 by the
Pilgrims' Friend Society,

175 Tower Bridge Road, London SE1 2AL.
Tel +44 0300 303 1400.

Email: info@pilgrimsfriend.org.uk
Website: www.pilgrimsfriend.org.uk

Distributed by the Pilgrims' Friend Society, London.

For just as the body is one and has many members, and all the members of the body, though many are one body, so it is with Christ. For in one Spirit we were all baptised into one body – Jews or Greeks, slaves or free – and all were made to drink of one, Spirit. For the body does not consist of one member but of many. If the foot should say, "Because I am not a hand I do not belong to the body," that would not make it any less a part of the body. And if the ear should say, "because I am not an eye, I do not belong to the body," that would not make it any less a part of the body. If the whole body were an eye, where would be the sense of hearing? If the whole body were an ear, where would be the sense of smell? But as it is, God arranged the members of the body, each one of them, as He chose. If all were a single member, where would the body be? As it is, there are many parts, yet one body.

If one member suffers, all suffer together: if one member is honoured, all rejoice together.

1 Corinthians 12

Contents

The importance of church for people with dementia

Church is central to the lives of Christians. Church means more to us than just attending a service on a Sunday; it's about fellowship and community, encouragement and support, enjoying the Scriptures, and growing in our faith. Both our church and faith are part of our identity.

In our talks and training on dementia with faith groups and churches, one of the questions we ask is 'what would you miss most if you were not able to go to church?' Most people have to think before answering, because church is so much a part of our lives that we have to step back and hold it at arm's length to see the detail. Some people say they would miss the ritual, some say the fellowship, some say the sermon, but most say, 'the corporate worship.' The songs, the hymns, the expressions of our love for Jesus.

Churches are more important for the wellbeing of Christians with dementia than most of us realise. The trailblazer in understanding dementia and promoting person-centred care, Professor Tom Kitwood wrote that 'Holding the person together is the main aim of good dementia care. Identity remains when others help to hold it in place.' He added that, 'When it comes to caring for someone with dementia, 'It might be said that there is only one all-encompassing need – for love.' (Dementia Reconsidered, OUP, 2011)

Being in church helps reinforce the person's sense of identity. The familiar liturgy, the fellowship of others – and the worship especially, reflect God's love. We know that music and singing have a powerful effect on the brain. On YouTube is a video of Henry, a man who had been unresponsive for over two years, apparently lost to the world, who came alive again listening to the jazz and Christian music that had been part of his life. (Google, Henry comes alive listening to music.) In the video, neurologist Oliver Sacks describes how music is a 'quickening art' and the effect lasts long after the music stops.

There is healing power for the soul in Christian worship. In one of his devotional books, Selwyn Hughes, one of Wales' best-loved preachers, pointed out that in worship we find unity, not just with God but within ourselves. He wrote,

'How do we get the framework, the sense of structure we need to be able to move effectively from one day to

another, in a world where everything that seemed to be nailed down is coming apart? It is to be found in our worship of God. We enter into the presence of the Lord and lo, His unity becomes our unity.'

More and more churches are keen to be 'dementia friendly'. We would like that to be moved forward to 'dementia inclusive,' or even, as one church member put it, 'dementia embracing'. Many people with dementia have said they would not like the term to be flagged up at all but for churches to simply *do it* and *be it.*

Good information and training are available from a number of sources, but they miss the most important element of all for Christians, that of *spiritual support*. We agree with the apostle Paul when he wrote to the Christians at Thessalonica that he prayed for their 'whole spirit and soul and body.' (1 Thessalonians 5:23). Good care and support, at any level, works best when it is holistic.

Church is also there for the wider community and for people who are not believers, including those with dementia. A woman we met at conference told us about her mother who had determinedly rejected the gospel and who had always been difficult; increasingly more so now she had developed dementia. When she said she was going to come to church with her next Sunday, the daughter was apprehensive, wondering how she would behave. She was surprisingly quiet and said she would like to go again next week. The following week she went and responded to the altar call, committing her life to the Lord. Dementia is no obstacle to the work of the Holy Spirit.

The purpose of this book is to give churches the information they need in order to become places where people with dementia and their families can go and feel comfortable, be strengthened in their faith and be supported in their personal pilgrimages.

* * *

For more information and to arrange for training go to info@pilgrimsfriend.org.uk, or to the website, www.pilgrimsfriend.org.uk, where you will find other resources for helping people with dementia and their families.

* * *

Can anything ever separate us from Christ's love? Does it mean he no longer loves us if we have trouble or calamity, or are persecuted, or hungry, or destitute, or in danger, or threatened with death?

And I am convinced that nothing can ever separate us from God's love. Neither death nor life, neither angels nor demons,[b] neither our fears for today nor our worries about tomorrow—not even the powers of hell can separate us from God's love. No power in the sky above or in the earth below—indeed, nothing in all creation will ever be able to separate us from the love of God that is revealed in Christ Jesus our Lord.

Romans 8: 35, 38.

About dementia

Dementia is a Latin word that means, literally, apart from or away from the mind. It is not a description of the disease itself but of the symptoms. There are many different causes of dementia, but in the simplest terms dementia results from physical damage to the brain. Among the main causes are Alzheimer's disease, Lewy body dementia, vascular infarct (strokes), Pick's disease, Posterior Cortical Atrophy, and Frontotemporal dementia. When we mention dementia, we are referring to the effects of the physical damage to the brain from these various causes.

The producers of the psychiatrists diagnostic handbook the DSM, the Diagnostic and Statistical Manual of Mental Disorders, refer to dementia as 'a neurological disorder' and would prefer to replace the term 'Dementia' with "major neurocognitive disorder and mild neurocognitive disorder". However they acknowledge that the disease will probably continue to be called 'Dementia', as the name has been widely adopted and is snappier to use.

In the last few years, observers comment that dementia has become 'Alzheimerised', with all forms swept into the Alzheimer's category. In 2019 An international team of researchers proposed a name for another type of brain disease that causes dementia symptoms: Limbic-predominant Age-related TDP-43 Encephalopathy, or LATE. The name is appropriate because it occurs mainly in older people. It causes problems similar to those seen in Alzheimer's disease and other types of dementia. It's thought to be caused by the protein, TDP-43, which is usually present in the centre of nerve cells but may change form and spread into the body of nerve cells as people get older. It's thought to affect around 20% of adults over 80. It is important to note that although dementia is more common in older people, it is not an inevitable part of ageing. It's most prevalent in those aged 80 and over.

The symptoms of dementia interfere with the person's daily activities. The symptoms can include (but are not limited to) forgetting events, names and places, repeating questions, difficulty finding words or putting thoughts in conversation, problems managing money, getting lost in familiar places, trouble doing work of routine tasks, depression, lethargy and apathy, neglecting appearance and personality changes. Diagnosis is made at a memory clinic, but it is not a straightforward process. Some people may have a condition known as mild cognitive impairment, or MCI, thought to be a precursor to dementia, although studies show that 70% of people fully recover in a 'nonclinical setting'. MCI can be caused by a number of conditions, including anaemia, poor diet, stress, feelings of loneliness, reactions to medication, urinary infection, and depression.

There is no cure for dementia but there are some medications that can help to hold back the progression. It's widely acknowledged that the best 'treatment' for people with dementia is the quality of care they receive.

There are many reported instances when people with dementia, often in quite deep dementia, seem to step through the fog and become lucid, with faculties that had assumed to be lost. It's a phenomenon known as 'rementing'.

It happens usually in response to a stimulus that is meaningful to the person. In our care homes it's observed in people taking part in daily devotions. One care home manager told of Winifred, singing a hymn with her face alive with meaning and joy. One of our pastoral volunteers, a former missionary and pastor tells how his attitude towards preaching to people with dementia completely changed after taking one of the services. A lady with deep dementia was wheeled in looking totally uncomprehending. Her eyes were blank and her jaw slack. She stayed like that until he opened the big Bible he uses for the services, and then her head came up, her mouth closed, and her eyes were fixed on him the entire time he read from it. It was clear to him that she understood what he was saying. When he had finished speaking her head drooped again and she was as before.

Professor Kitwood noted that 'A study of homes where the care was of very high quality found clear examples of 'rementing', a measurable recovery of powers that had apparently been lost. (Dementia Reconsidered.) As well as having care of a very high quality, Pilgrims' Friend Society's homes have a Christian ethos and practice.

In the book, *Dementia: Pathways to Hope*, Louise Morse quotes Psalm 42, and the famous book by Chinese Pastor Watchman Nee, 'Deep calls to Deep', and reasons that even when other faculties have failed the Holy Spirit can communicate directly to the spirit of the person. Watchman Nee wrote, 'nothing shallow can ever touch the depths, nor can anything superficial touch the inward parts. Only the deep will respond to the deep. Anything that does not issue from the depths cannot touch the depths.'

* * *

If you love me, keep my commands. And I will ask the Father, and he will give you another advocate to help you and be with you forever – the Spirit of truth. The world cannot accept him, because it neither sees him nor knows him. But you know him, for he lives with you and will be in you. I will not leave you as orphans; I will come to you.

John 14: 25, 16 (NASB)

Laying the groundwork

We are usually asked to give talks and train in churches when some of the members begin to develop dementia. They will be people who are known to the fellowship and are familiar with its routines and the building. Other churches ask because they want to be prepared and understand what dementia is, what to expect, what sort of support they can give and how best to provide it. Beginning with page 25 we describe the six key steps to making a truly inclusive dementia church. They cover practical, psychological and spiritual aspects.

But even before beginning the process it's important to understand as much as possible about dementia and how it affects people living with it and their families. Most people know very little about dementia, even when their lives are affected by it, and there are still many myths and misunderstandings.

Sometimes we hear people ask, 'what's the point of bothering with someone with dementia? They don't understand what you're saying, and they don't remember who you are.'

The truth is that when people seem to be unresponsive and shut away inside themselves, there is often more going on in their minds than we realise. In the book, 'Dementia from the Inside, a Doctor's Personal Journey of Hope' (Bute and Morse, 2018, SPCK), Jennifer Bute, a GP diagnosed with dementia in 2009, tells how people with dementia can be brought into the present, and even learn to speak again. Although the effects of the disease seem to change an individual's personality, specialists know that the person remains.

Christine Bryden was a top executive with the Australian Government when she was diagnosed with Young Onset Dementia at the age of 49. She became a voice for people with dementia, writing and speaking at international conferences. Speaking at a conference in New Zealand in 2005, she entreated:

'As I lose an identity in the world around me,

which is so anxious to define me by what I do and say, rather than who I am,

I can seek an identity by simply being me, a person created in the image of God.

My spiritual self is reflected in the divine and given meaning as a transcendent being.

As I travel toward the dissolution of myself, my personality, my very 'essence', my relationship with God needs increasing support from you, my other in the body of Christ.

Don't abandon me at any stage, for the Holy Spirit connects us. …I need you to minister to me, to sing with me, pray with me, to be my memory for me …

You play a vital role in relating to the soul within me, connecting at this eternal level.

Sing alongside me, touch me, pray with me, and reassure me of your presence,

and through you, of Christ's presence.

I need you to be the Christ-light for me, to affirm my identity and walk alongside me.'

'In another context she added,

'I may not be able to affirm you, to remember who you are or whether you visited me. But you have brought Christ

to me. If I enjoy your visit, why must I remember it? Why must I remember who you are? Is this just to satisfy your own need for identity? So please allow Christ to work through you. Let me live in the present. If I forget a pleasant memory, it does not mean that it was not important for me.'

* * *

Every Sunday morning, 87-year-old Kenneth is collected with a few others by minibus from his care home in the Suffolk country side and taken to church. The minibus collects others from their own homes, too. Care home staff had been a little concerned that Kenneth, who has dementia, might 'leg it', as they put it, because suddenly and without warning, he would decide to go for a walk, loping at incredible speed across the fields that he knows so well in the Suffolk countryside. No matter how dementia friendly the church, would he be bored and 'do a runner'?

They needn't have worried. At church Kenneth was paired up with a 'buddy'; someone he knew who would befriend him, sit alongside him and make sure that he had everything he needed. It turns out that Kenneth is so contented in church that he has never shown the slightest inclination to 'leg it', to everyone's relief. He sits throughout the service, joining in when a snatch of a hymn stirs his memory, and occasionally falling asleep on his buddy's shoulder during the sermon. If he becomes restless at any point his buddy will take him to the toilet, or offer him a drink from the kitchen, or even walk with him around the church garden before going back inside. But most of the time Kenneth sits, listens, zones in and out and oozes contentment. He's been a Christian for most of his life and simply being in church, with its liturgy and the hymns he'd always loved, and its sense of peace was like being at home. It resonated with the life-long practices and the beliefs at the core of his being: and in that comfortable, long-known environment, the Holy Spirit ministers to his soul. What's true of Kenneth can also be said of the others with dementia in the congregation.

For believers, our church fellowship is our central, core community. It's where we learn, share, make friendships, and find encouragement and support. It's where we worship; where in the truest sense we are known and accepted. But sadly, most people with dementia stop going to church. They feel uncomfortable, not because their church has changed but because their ability to process information is impaired. They can't quite 'compute' what is going on; they forget names and faces and have sudden 'blanks', and feel vulnerable outside their own four walls, so they withdraw to the safety of their own homes, where they will not be confronted with these alarming 'blanks'. Kenneth's church didn't want that to happen, and a few years ago began a process that has led to it becoming a truly dementia inclusive church. 'Dementia friendly' is rather a weak description – 'dementia embracing' describes it better.

Everyone at Kenneth's church has been trained in understanding dementia, including what to expect and how to respond. This is important, as people with dementia can behave in unexpected ways. In Kenneth's church seating for people with dementia, and for those in wheelchairs is arranged at the back so they can leave and return without causing a disturbance. On one occasion Betty decided she wanted to inspect the visiting preacher more closely, and leaving her chair she walked up the aisle and stood in front of him, peering at him intently. He moved to one side so that he could see the congregation, but Betty moved as well, so he moved to the other side and she followed there. At that point her 'buddy' caught up with her and slipping her arm through hers led her away saying, 'let's go now and have a cup of tea.'

In a church in America Sam was sitting with his daughter. She'd tried a few local churches, but they seemed uncomfortable with her father. She hoped that this church would be more accepting, and so far, it was going well. The pastor was preaching on the concept of life being a pilgrimage, a journey on our way to Heaven. 'We are all on our way Home,' he said. At which point Sam shouted, 'Home, Home on the Range!' Without missing a beat the pastor turned to the music group and asked, 'Can we play that one?' They could, and the whole church joined in singing 'Home, Home on the Range!' Both Sam and his daughter knew that the Lord had brought them to the right church.

We are not to confuse holiness with the predictability or the order of the service. In recent years the introduction of 'messy church' has led to more acceptance of things that contribute in a different way. Many congregations have become more understanding of people with dementia, and more accepting.

* * *

"For the Lord does not see as man sees:
for man looks at the outward appearance,
but the Lord looks at the heart."

1 Samuel 16:7

Six key steps to creating a dementia friendly church

Step one – having the full commitment of the pastoral team and the empathy of an informed congregation.

It is essential to have the full support and commitment of the pastoral team. These are the members who are responsible for addressing issues within the church through regular preaching and teaching. They will bring the vision to the fellowship, and at the same time in understanding about the condition itself. The surge in the prevalence of dementia has brought to everyone's attention a condition that is unfamiliar to most.

Before teaching about dementia there will have been exposition of Christ's compassion and the imperative of caring for one another. Applying Scriptural precepts to our lives provides the framework and the desire to create safe, caring fellowships where vulnerable people with dementia find acceptance. There will have been a background of pastoral teaching on the value of each person to God, and how each one, including those with dementia is made in His image. Each Christian with dementia has an immortal soul and is precious in the sight of God: as part of the body of Christ should receive ministry from their local church as they journey along their dementia pathway.

The keys to Step One are:

1. obtaining everyone's commitment to the concept of dementia friendly church

2. pastoral leaders taking a key role

3. acknowledging that every human being is made in God's image

4. caring for one another is commanded in the Scriptures, and indeed, precious to Christ (Matthew 25:40)

Step two – Making the building dementia friendly

Many dementias involve visual problems. These include difficulty in distinguishing between colours and textures, the loss of peripheral vision and not being able to see things on either side, not being able to judge distance or depth, and the ability to interpret an image. Here are a few pointers to making your church building easier to navigate and safer, not just for people with dementia but also for older people whose vision may be affected.

- ensure that there is good lighting everywhere.

- avoid mirrors. Even in toilets.

- provide good signage, using images as well as words where possible.

- in toilets, use contrasting colours – for example, if the walls are white, red or green for the lavatory seat.

- avoid shiny floors which will appear wet to those with dementia

- also avoid strongly patterned flooring which can be confusing

- light-coloured flooring is better than dark

- avoid using blue/grey tones – warm tones are seen more easily

- don't have 'slip rugs'

- don't have seating which is the same colour or tone as the flooring

- dark thresholds in a doorway may appear as a hole or barrier, and a black or very dark mat may appear to be a hole

- different floorings laid adjacent to each other should blend together so as not to create the appearance of a step

- where there are steps, the edges need to be clearly seen, using fluorescent tape along the edge or something similar to highlight them

- as far as possible, ensure that each space has good tonal contrast between floors, walls and doors

- if the church has a coffee shop or eating area using white crockery, don't use white-topped tables. Use a strong colour so that people with dementia can see easily the boundaries of their plates or saucers.

Step three – Identifying project leader(s) who share the vision

Pastors and church leaders need to identify members who have a vision for the dementia friendly work. Often in church fellowships there are occupational therapists or nurses or people in the caring profession who are happy to take ownership of the project. They can be the ones who will help train and support the rest of the church. They can start encouraging others with training and talks and presentations. Pilgrims' Friend Society's speakers are happy to become involved, and there are also excellent books and a Dementia Information Pack with separate inserts on our website, www.pilgrimsfriend.org.uk 'Visiting a Person with Dementia' is example.

Step four – Finding volunteers who are happy to be 'buddies' for people with dementia

Each case of dementia is unique, a combination of the disease and the individual's personality. Each person has had different life experiences that have left them with different expectations. Most often the person with dementia will come to church with a companion, but this is not always the case. In a small fellowship the person may know others that he or she is comfortable with, and they can sit together. It is important that people with dementia feel that there is someone close who can help when needed. It may be a small thing, such as answering a question, or going out with the person if necessary. In a larger church 'buddies' can be a great comfort sitting alongside an individual, or a couple. In the case of the daughter whose mother came with her to church for the first time, a friendly individual alongside helped put her at her ease. In another instance, a nephew would take his aunt to church and leave her at the door, as he had no interest in church himself. Each circumstance is different but having people ready to sit alongside can be invaluable.

Step five – Understanding how to communicate

Understanding and communicating with people with dementia is paramount. Learning how to do this strengthens our communications with others, too. Here are some golden rules.

- Don't greet the person from the back with a tap on the shoulder. Always greet them from the front.

- Always smile warmly and make eye contact.

- Don't stand over the person but sit alongside.

- Speak clearly, and not too fast. On the other hand don't speak too slowly or the person may feel you are cross with them. Don't say too much at once.

- Each person with dementia is different, but don't ask questions that involve recalling memories or working things out. Ask questions only that are relevant in the moment, such as 'how are you feeling today?' or, 'are you comfortable sitting here?'

- Don't interrupt the person and don't contradict, even if he says something which you know is not correct. For example, if an 80-year-old says her mother will be coming in a short while, you can deflect by saying something enthusiastic or relevant such as 'what a blessing mothers are! Where would we be without them! Now my mother ...' Always deflect empathetically. There used to be a technique called 'Reality Orientation', but it is accepted now that a) it can be shocking and harmful to the person to be confronted in this way and b) keeping the person emotionally balanced is more important. It is the disease and not the person.

- Sometimes it's necessary to look for the emotions behind what the person is saying. For example, if someone says, 'I want to go home' it can mean that they're not feeling comfortable and not feeling at ease. Finding out what you can do to make the person feel at ease may answer the need. Sometimes just having a cup of tea in the kitchen before returning may be all it takes.

- A person with dementia may think they are speaking logically but often their words are scrambled. Try to identify the emotion, or the meaning.

Sometimes the situation gives you a clue, or their body language.

- People with dementia can repeat things. But if they do, don't tell them that they have just said that. Repetition can be a sign that the person wants to make contact with you.

- Be mindful about your body language: positive facial expressions and a relaxed posture will say more than words can convey. A person with dementia will understand the emotions you are expressing more than the words you are using. Sometimes 'being' is far more important than 'doing', so use touch and gestures appropriately to express emotion.

Step 6 – regular assessments, prayer meetings, and staying in touch

Prayer for people with dementia and their families should be a normal part of church activity, and it is good to have regular meetings with the dementia team leaders and with others who are interested to discuss how it is working, and how it could be improved. There are often new suggestions in the light of experience. It's important to reflect on what is working well and what needs to improve. Where people come with family members or with friends it's a good idea to ask them how they feel it is working. They may have suggestions that could help.

Not forgetting caregivers

Many churches hold regular meetings for people with dementia and their caregivers. Others have separate meetings for caregivers, including for those after their role has ended, when their care recipient has died.

But it often happens that as the illness progresses the person with dementia finds leaving the home too disturbing. At home they feel safe and are not confronted with cognitive 'blanks' and memory lapses. Over time the caregiver, usually a spouse or adult child, withdraws with them, in a syndrome known as 'role entrapment'.

Eventually they slip off the church's radar and are forgotten – at the very time they need more support than ever. The team looking after the dementia friendly church programme should keep in touch with them. By now they should have an idea of what support the family needs, but if not, they can ask, or simply give a telephone number to contact when a need arises. There are a lot of practical things that would be welcome, such as a little help with the garden, being on hand for changing a lightbulb, collecting a prescription or taking over a cooked meal now and then.

Most importantly, pastor leaders and others should let the family know that they are not forgotten, and that they are still remembered in prayer. When the main caregiver needs someone to talk to, or even pray with, a telephone number and a person they can call will make a big difference to them. Even just knowing it is available is a reasssurance and comfort.

This does not need to be the sole responsibility of the dementia team leader(s).

Many people in a fellowship are willing to offer a little time, and share their talents. They can let the leaders know the times that they are available and what they can do. A well-run support project can be literally, life-saving for caregivers. Research shows that dementia caregiver burden causes ill health, and in older spouses can lead to them developing dementia themselves or an early death.

* * *

'The King will reply, 'Truly I tell you, whatever you did for one of the least of these brothers and sisters of mine, you did for me.'

Matthew 25: 40

Talks and seminars:
Available from the Pilgrims' Friend Society:

1. Making a truly dementia friendly church

2. Dementia – practical and spiritual insights

3. Dementia – the support and help that churches can give

4. Early dementia and the vital circles of support

5. Visiting people with dementia

6. Giving effective support to family caregivers

7. Empowering and engaging older people

8. How churches can effectively support dementia families

9.   Caregivers – how to care for yourselves

10. Ministering in care homes

11. Dealing with loneliness

12. How to prepare for a great old age

13. Developing your talents and gifting after retirement

14. Empowering older people

15. Caring for parents and other older relatives

16. Building communities, a street at a time

17. Christians and retirement

18. End of life care, and what matters in the end.

19. Legal issues in old age

20. What to expect from domiciliary care

21. When a care home is best

Recommended reading

Dementia: Pathways to Hope
Louise Morse

Published by Lion Monarch, November 2015

'Dementia is having an impact on people of all ages, not just the elderly. Families, friends and church fellowships are all being affected. Louise's 'pathways to hope' highlights the importance of guarding the heart, and of being strengthened in our spirits for whatever life brings us, whether or not it includes dementia. This book contains much helpful information and is enlightening and encouraging: it will help individuals and churches alike.'

Clyde Thomas,
Senior Pastor, Victory Church, Cwmbran, South Wales.

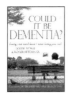

Could it be Dementia

Louise Morse and Roger Hitchings

Published by Lion Monarch, 978 0 8254 6170 5

'This book inspires on so many levels – to the carer for whom it is a resource, full of ideas and memory-joggers – but most of all, to the dementia sufferer, because it might provide the key to unlock the soul of a Christian whose mind has forgotten the loving God their heart has always known and longed for.'

Pam Rhodes, TV presenter

DEMENTIA:
Frank and Linda's Story

Louise Morse

Published by Lion Monarch, 978-1-85424-930-2

'Firmly rooted in the sanctity of 'God's image', replete with practical advice and useful links, this is a resource for individual caregivers, health professionals, church families, and all thinking Christians.'

Dr Cameron Swift, consultant physician and Professor of Healthcare of the Elderly

'The best book for understanding the dementia journey,'

Dr Jennifer Bute.

Worshipping with Dementia

Louise Morse

Published by Lion Monarch, 978-1-85424-931-9

Meditations, Scriptures and Prayers for people coping with dementia 'This is so helpful to me and my team visiting our local care homes.'

Team of retired Vicar and colleagues.

Helping to Put the Pieces Together

An information pack produced by the Pilgrims' Friend Society, with separate inserts on different aspects of dementia.

'Your user-friendly pack has made me feel at peace and confident that I will be able to cope, either with getting dementia myself or becoming a carer.'

Joy Watson

Contended Dementia

Oliver James

Published by Vermillion, ISBN 1407028871

Describes the SPECAL method of relational care themed over 30 years by Penny Garner; recommended by the Royal College of Nurses.

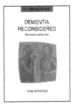

Dementia Reconsidered

Tom Kitwood

Published by Open University Press, ISBN 0-335-19855-4

A seminal work with many reprints by the late Professor Kitwood of Bradford University. Tom Kitwood revolutionised the care of people with dementia.

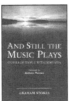

And Still The Music Plays

Graham Stokes

Published by Hawker Publications, ISBN 978-1874790952

A small book, written with expertise and compassion, showing how people with dementia behave according to their intrinsic values and beliefs.

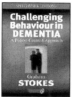

Challenging Behaviour in Dementia

Graham Stokes

Published by Speechmark Publishing, ISBN: 9780863883972

Written mainly for health care professionals, Dr. Stokes' book explains the possible reasons behind challenging behaviour and the best ways of understanding and coping with it.

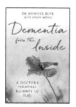

Dementia From the Inside

Dr Jennifer Bute

with Louise Morse

Published by SPCK Publishing, 978-0-28108-069-4

Many assume that living with dementia is one long term steady decline. Jennifer's insightful book debunks that myth.

Jeremy Hughes, Chief Executive, Alzheimer's Society

www.gloriousopportunity.org

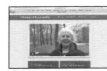 Valuable practical and spiritual insights by Dr Jennifer Bute, a general practitioner diagnosed with early onset dementia.

Dr Bute shares medical and personal insights into dementia, and her website has a wealth of valuable information.

Organisations that can help:

Here is a selection of organisations that are geared up to helping you.

1. **Age UK** (formerly Age Concern and Help The Aged) – the UK's largest charity working with and for older people, with links to local branches.

    Tel: 0800 169 6565;

    Web: www.ageuk.org.uk

2. **Alzheimer's Society** – the UK's leading care and research charity for people with dementia and their carers.

    Tel: 0845 300 0336;

    Web: www.alzheimers.org.uk

3. **Care Quality Commission** – website shows rating for UK care homes.

   Tel: 03000 616161

   Web: www.cqc.org.uk

4. **Carers Allowance Unit** – part of Department of Work and Pensions, giving advice on the Carer's Allowance, the main state benefit for carers.

   Tel: 0845 608 4321;

   Text Phone: 0845 604 5312

   Web: www.direct.gov.uk/carers-allowance

5. **Carers' Christian Fellowship** – offers mutual support, sharing and prayer.

   Tel: 023 8028 3270;

   Web: www.carerschristianfellowship.org

6. **Carers UK** – offers support with caring for carers.

   Tel: 0808 808 7777;

   Web: www.carersuk.org

7. **Counsel and Care** (for older people, their families and carers) – provides personalized and in-depth advice.

    Tel: 0845 300 7585;

    Web: www.counselandcare.org.uk

8. **Brunel Care** (incorporating Dementia Care Trust) – offers accommodation, health care, counselling and other assistance, to prolong an independent lifestyle.

    Tel: 0117 914 4200;

    Web: www.brunelcare.org.uk

9. **Dementia UK** – offering practical advice and emotional support to people affected by dementia through fully trained Admiral Nurses

    Tel: 020 7874 7200;

    Web: www.dementiauk.org

    Admiral Nursing Direct: 0845 257 9406

10. **Dementia Web** (formerly DISC) – an all-age dementia information resource for the UK, providing information about other related services across the UK

    Tel: 0845 120 4048;

    Web: www.dementiaweb.org.uk

11. **Tourism For All** – charity specialising in accessible holiday and respite services for older and disabled people and their carers (helps make tourism welcoming to all).

    Tel: 0845 124 9971;

    Web: www.tourismforall.org.uk

12. **Office of the Public Guardian** – helps with planning for one's future.

    Tel: 0300 456 0300;

    Web: www.publicguardian.gov.uk

13. **PARCHE** – Pastoral Action in Residential Care Homes for the Elderly; training for church teams.

    Tel: 01323 438527;

    Web: www.parche.org.uk

14. **Parish Nursing Ministries UK** – whole person health care through the local church.

    Tel: 01788 817904;

    Web: www.parishnursing.org.uk

15. **The Frontotemporal Dementia Support Group** (incorporating Pick's Disease Support Group) – caring for people with Frontotemporal dementia, with regional links.

    Web: www.ftdsg.org

16. **Relatives and Residents Association** – information about residential care and help if things go wrong.

    Tel: 020 7359 8136;

    Web: www.relres.org

17. **Contented Dementia Trust** (formerly SPECAL) – dementia charity providing courses, services and advice. Is known best for its themed approach to care.

    Web: www.contenteddementiatrust.org

18. **Carers Trust** (formerly Princess Royal Trust and Crossroads Care) – works to improve carers' services and helps carers make their needs and voices heard.

    Tel: 0844 800 4361

    Web: www.carers.org

19. **Independent Age** – advice and information on home care, care homes, going into hospital and related issues.

    Tel: 0845 262 1863

    Web: www.independentage.org

20. **AT Dementia** – Information on assistive technology for people with dementia.

    Tel: 0116 257 5017

    Web: www.atdementia.org.uk

21. **Guideposts Trust** – provides direct services to people with dementia, their families and carers, to help them make the best choice for care services.

    Tel: 01993 772886;

    Web: www.guidepoststrust.org.uk

22. **Alzheimer's Research UK** – provides information on the different types of dementia, their symptoms and the treatments available to help.

    Tel: 01223 843899

    Web: www.alzheimersresearchuk.org

International

23. **Age International** – helps older people in developing countries by reducing poverty, improving health, protecting rights and responding to emergencies.

    Web: www.ageinternational.org.uk

More books from
Pilgrims' Friend Society

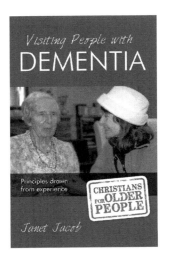

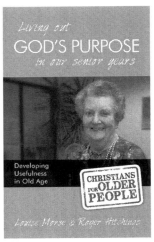

Visiting People With Dementia

978 0 9930 1481 9

Living Out God's Purpose in Our Senior Years

978 0 9930 1483 3

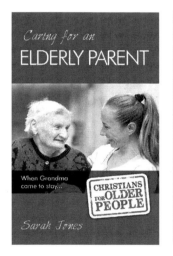

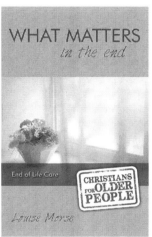

**Caring for an
Elderly Parent**

978 0 9930 1487 1

**What Matters
in the End**

978 0 9930 1489 5